CHANGE MADE EASY
NUTRIENT-LESS TO NUTRIENT-RICH

KELLY FONTAMILLAS

Special thank you to mom, dad, sister, hubs, boo, and the bubs; Amy, Duane, Kristi, Jeni, Joy, Wayne, & Wendy. You have all contributed to this book in more ways than you know.

CONTENTS

1. INTRODUCTION

The purpose of this book is to make it easier for us to change the way we eat because America makes it so hard. We're not informed enough about what we are consuming, and since we don't see negative effects on our health immediately, we just blame age or genetics. It seems so obvious that what we feed our bodies has a lot to do with many of our physical and mental sufferings, but for some reason we don't think about that. We may consider the calories, but we care most about the taste, and it's no secret that health food has a bad rap for flavor. This book will set your mind up for change and how to do it gradually so it's not overwhelming. Plus, change is way easier when recipes are already created for you that taste like you haven't changed anything. The recipes included mimic the taste of the real sugary and overly processed foods we love, but no one will know that my sweet treats are low-no sugar, wheat-free, dairy-free, and soy-free. But, first, let me begin by telling what made me change in the first place. I was just a regular girl with a serious sweet tooth, and some mild, but annoying, health issues seemingly completely unrelated to food. Join me as my story unfolds and see for yourself how the food we eat is wreaking havoc on our bodies unaware.

2. JOURNEY

The seed was planted when I was a little girl standing in the freezer aisle of a grocery store with my mom. We went there to get frozen whipped topping because it was less fattening than whipped cream. I remember inquiring about how it was made without dairy. My mom replied something about "chemicals." I was skeptical, but shrugged it off. Later, while standing in the checkout line, my mom bought a pack of artificially sweetened gum like she frequently did. I remember reading the label which said something about causing cancer in laboratory mice. When I questioned it, my mom's exact words were, "Oh, we can never eat as much as they give to mice." I was still skeptical, but shrugged it off again because I honestly thought that if it was sold to us it couldn't be that bad.

That little seed didn't sprout until about fifteen years later when I grabbed a soda from the vending machine in between classes in college and read the ingredients out of boredom, *"Brominated vegetable oil? What is that?"* I asked aloud. A classmate responded, suggesting it was something that is used in pools, or something that is poisonous in a solid form. I furrowed my brow in suspicion of what else was put in our food, and was reminded of that naïve little girl standing in the freezer aisle buying something not natural. For the first time, I realized that I was not informed enough about what I was feeding the cells of my body. I had to look out for myself because I couldn't trust what was put on the shelves of our markets anymore.

Trans Fat & PHO (partially hydrogenated oils)

If you asked me in college if I thought I was a healthy eater, I would have answered, "yes." I ate my share of fruits and vegetables; stayed away from red meat most of the time, and exercised regularly. I didn't exactly know why candy and junk food was bad for *me,* a girl who had to have her size zero wedding dress taken in. I didn't think I was at risk for diabetes or obesity. I ate whatever I wanted to, and, boy, did I have a sweet tooth. I admit that once in a while I would eat dessert for dinner, but made sure I ate a big salad the next day. The thought of going without something sweet for a day was absurd, which is why I sipped on my favorite Thai Iced-tea almost daily. I enjoyed baking, so I made anything I ever wanted to on a whim. I didn't think my diet needed any changing.

When I decided that I should scrutinize food labels, I became aware of the ingredients in the packaged food I was eating. I started wondering about all the hydrogenated oils I was seeing. Soon after, I heard a blurb on TV about the dreadful terms "trans fat," "hydrogenated oil," and "shortening." It was reported that shortening was a trans fat because it was hydrogenated oil, which was not good for our hearts, and other organs. I quickly regretted that I ate French fries almost every day for nine years when I worked at Burger King. After all, everyone said vegetable shortening was better than lard and other oils known to have saturated fat, like coconut oil. I also carry around guilt over that time I convinced an elderly man, who "really wanted French fries," to just give in because they were fried in vegetable shortening, not lard. The vegetable oil was still attacking our hearts even without the cholesterol. (Many restaurants have since changed their oils, but read on to learn why the non-hydrogenated oils are not much better.)

Unexpectedly, one day, a friend approached me regarding a book he was reading called, *The Coconut Oil Miracle* (Fife, 2004). I was interested in what my friend said, so I bought the book and appreciated how it taught me about fats and oils on a molecular level, and why certain oils with saturated fat are healthier than others. I grew up in the era when everyone said that all saturated fat was bad for us. We were cooking with shortening and eating margarine because the soybean industry created a solid unsaturated fat by manually adding hydrogen atoms to a liquid oil to make a solid (e.g., shortening), producing *partially hydrogenated oil*. Using shortening in place of butter and lard seemed like a great idea because it was thought to be healthier and also acted as a preservative increasing the shelf life of boxed goods. It appeared to be the perfect frying oil sans cholesterol. It was an ideal ingredient for food manufacturers, so just about the whole world switched to this alleged healthier oil, and it was very affordable. We ate it thinking it was good for us. The problem was, instead of being a saturated fat, it was now a trans fatty acid (aka trans fat), which we now know that our bodies can't effectively process causing free radical cells to form destroying the healthy ones. Fife, the author, explains that as we ingest trans fat our cells steal electrons away from other healthy ones forming the free radical cells. Research has linked free radical cell damage to heart disease, cancer, atherosclerosis, stroke, varicose veins, hemorrhoids, high blood pressure, wrinkles, dermatitis, arthritis, digestive problems, reproductive problems, cataracts, loss of energy, diabetes, allergies, and memory loss (Fife, 2004). In addition, unsaturated, non-hydrogenated oils, like canola, soybean, and olive oil, oxidize quickly (think of rust on metal) when processed, heated, and exposed to light, causing free radical cells to form within our bodies when we eat it. (Olive oil should be used after cooking like in pastas and dressings.) Trans fat and oxidized oil changes and damages our cells. So, after reading *The Coconut Oil Miracle*, I was motivated to eliminate trans fat from my diet and to eat more antioxidant rich food to help repair the damage I had done from all the cell oxidation. I did not know, however, that trans fat was going to be hidden in just about everything I ate.

I spent hours in the aisles of supermarkets reading every ingredient in most packaged foods to see if it had *partially hydrogenated oil* listed.

You have to look beyond the nutritional label. I found it hidden in everything I ate and grew up eating. It was in all name brand cookies (some have since taken it out, supposedly), all cake and brownie mixes, frosting, the majority of crackers, candy bars, refrigerated dough, milk substitute products (including frozen whipped topping), flavored dairy creamers, some peanut butters, hot chocolate mixes, dip mixes, cheaper brands of chocolates; margarines, breads, tortillas, cereals, pastries, pie crust, frozen dinners, and even packaged and canned soup. The list went on and on. I wandered around the aisles wondering what I could then eat. I knew I had to start eating whole food. I just didn't really know where to start. I kept telling myself, *"Think back to the farm"* and *"What did Adam and Eve eat?"* I had already chucked my margarine at home, so bought some real butter. I bought a few things that I knew were good for me and full of antioxidants, such as berries and dark leafy greens and more vegetables that replaced the processed stuff. My cells had a lot of repairing to do.

After all that time spent reading labels, I knew what stuff would likely contain trans fats, so it was easy to avoid eating various things when I was at a restaurant or at a holiday party laden with sweet treats. My mouth used to water at the sight of a specific brand of doughnuts, but, instead, they just disgusted me. I avoided cravings by telling myself that they were tainted with poison slowing destroying my body. I vowed that I would never knowingly eat anything with partially hydrogenated oil again (aka trans fat). I cared about the health of my cells too much.

The Food and Drug Administration (FDA) allows .5 grams or less trans fat within a product to be counted as zero on the nutritional label. It is unknown how honest the food companies are. Some pastry companies list 9 grams trans fat per serving, but another brand of similar pastry lists zero; both are made with partially hydrogenated vegetable oil. Even still, one serving of one food with .5 grams trans fat eaten three times a day would add up to be just too much.

When I shared my great discovery and new passion for boycotting so many foods, people rolled their eyes at me, my mom included. Some shrugged me off by saying that they only eat certain foods *"in moderation"* anyway. How much is *in moderation*? What it is for you is not the same as what it is for me. I would not want to consume something with partially hydrogenated oil "in moderation" because it's too harmful to ever have at all, in my opinion. People know trans fat is bad for us, but not many can explain the type of damage it does to our cells and the consequences that follow. If you saw on the menu board next to the calorie count "contains hidden trans fat that is known to cause cellular damage" you may change your mind. If everyone knew what it actually does to our cellular health then they may be more open for change. Telling others that it's "bad" for us is not as effective as explaining how free radical cells form causing common diseases. Others I told seemed interested, but not as eager to change what they ate because it was so hard, and I got the "oh-but- I- can't-live-without" complaint. Or, the "it's just one cookie. It's not going to kill me." True, it won't kill you, but your health will deteriorate much faster because it's not just one cookie. It's also the cereal you ate for breakfast, the bread in your sandwich at lunch, the crackers for snack, and the biscuit you had alongside dinner. And then, it is that one cookie. Then, it is the arthritis, the heart disease, and all the other health problems we don't typically relate to our food intake.

Change does not mean you have to go without. You have to find a healthier substitution, which is out there. I started making simple suggestions to people, including switching to a trans fat free margarine, such as the brand Earth Balance (organic or soy free varieties), and using real butter instead of shortening. Over time, I noticed my mom started making changes, too. She started by replacing her powdery nondairy creamer with a trans fat free milk powder. I was elated that someone I loved was up for the change. I suggested to others to start changing out one thing at a time to avoid being overwhelmed, such as just buying the trans fat free margarine and worrying about the bread they were eating later. I told people to continue to eat their favorite *Tater Tot Casserole* (baked with tater tots, cheese, mushroom soup) but to make their own cream of mushroom soup and to continue to use the tater tots fried in soybean oil for now (remember that oil oxidizes quickly when heated). It's really not that hard to make your own healthy versions of processed food; you just have to plan ahead. I made the soup a day before, froze half of it for later, and assembled the rest of the casserole the next day. Later, once you're established in avoiding trans fat, you'll consider shredding your own potatoes for the casserole, but let's just start with one thing at a time here. Sure it takes more effort than opening a can or bag, but it's totally worth it knowing your cells aren't being ripped apart.

The FDA recognizes that trans fat is not safe for consumption (FDA.gov) and is currently allowing a three year compliance period for food companies to phase out the use of partially hydrogenated oils. However, the type of oil they will likely replace with may be equally scary (more on that later). It's not just the oil that needs to be changed in our American diets anyway. It certainly wasn't for me...

Sugar

So how did I feed my sweet tooth since buying junk food at the supermarket was out of the question? I baked my own stuff. I made my own pie crusts with butter and chose recipes without shortening, for example. I was baking a goody every week, which were all trans fat free so I could still be satisfied. I did that until the day I learned that sugar was worse for me than I ever imagined. Why didn't anyone tell me all of this before? Was it new information or something?

It was during graduate school that I begun to learn how sugar directly affected me, which became clear to me in the years that followed. I was drinking more coffee than ever, sweetened with sugar, of course. I was too skeptical of the pink, blue, and yellow artificial packaged sweeteners that are sold to us. I began to feel like I was always in a fog. I was low on energy the majority of the time, so I drank more coffee thinking that would help. Instead, it seemed to make me slip into a cloudier fog; I never felt refreshed or alert and needed naps. Plus, I was really moody. So, naturally, I blamed it on the caffeine. I tried switching to tea sweetened with sugar, but then I started having disturbing bizarre dreams, so I blamed the caffeine in the tea again. I had a list of other ailments at that time, such as central dysacusis (i.e., overly sensitive hearing that makes loud noise painful), and, only in my twenties, I had to wrap my knee at night during the winter because it ached. A year after grad school my husband and I were planning for a family, so I weaned myself off of caffeine completely and the fog was lifted, but I still had the other issues (e.g., low energy, aching joint, sensitive hearing).

A few months after baby was born, my mom was diagnosed with stage IV breast cancer. There was no history of breast cancer in her family. Her mother had type II diabetes, not cancer. My mom went through hormone therapy during a period in her life, which may have contributed to her diagnosis. In addition, I was convinced that her diet along with the added stress at work before she retired had something to do with it. Did you know that our bodies successfully fight off cancer throughout our lifetime? That is until it does not fight off cancer. Tax the system with poor diet and stress we are bound to get something. It's a matter of *when,* not *if.* I want my *when* to be never. Genetics, of course, has a significant influence on what type of health issues we may face, which is why it is particularly important to change what we are consuming. Since my mom's diagnosis, I read a lot about the influence of food and nutrition on our bodies, specifically sugar, and turned to dear friends, who are health gurus, for advice. Did anyone ever tell you that sugar (i.e., glucose) directly feeds tumor cells making them grow much more rapidly? No one ever told me and I felt betrayed. Had my family known this growing up we would have likely maintained better diets. Combined with all of the trans fat America was eating I wasn't surprised at all of our autoimmune disorders anymore. It just depends on how our specific genetic makeup reacts to what we feed our cells and the stress of daily living. Will I get cancer, have a stroke, or age more rapidly? I learned that I was at risk for all of the above and more. I was sure I didn't want any of those things. I had to significantly reduce my sugar intake. I cringed at the sight of families loading up their carts with sodas, packaged foods, chips, cookies, and seemingly innocent items such as crackers and cereals knowing that it was laden with trans fat and sugar combined. Would they change if they knew *why* that stuff is bad? I did, so somebody else might, too. It's not junk food, it's garbage, literally littering our bodies, destroying and changing our systems. It's seems so obvious that what we feed our bodies causes cellular destruction and death, or cellular promotion, but for some reason it was not obvious to me until I read about how food actually changes our cells. "You have aching joints?" the doctor asks, and responds, "There is a medication for that." How about saying, "Let's also see how changing what you eat can help relieve those aching joints."

Sugar breaks down into our bodies as glucose. Our organs need glucose in order to function properly, like our brain, for one. But America gets too much glucose from drinking overpriced coffee and chugging sodas all day. I bought them thinking I was just buying something that tasted good. I knew they weren't doing anything good for me, but I never actually thought they were harming me. Part of the problem with America is that we are so busy we don't have the time to eat right, much less work out as often as we should. The first things to go in a busy life that gets even busier is your diet (drive through takes three minutes) and your cardio exercise because you would rather use that time to clean your house or actually sit down to unwind and enjoy a show. We don't want glucose sitting in our blood all day if we aren't burning it off through exercise. We certainly don't want glucose sitting in our blood all night when we are not active. I knew there was a good reason why I always wanted dessert before dinner or for breakfast! All cellular energy comes from glucose, but what happens to our cells when they are loaded with too much? They can't do their job. Nutrients aren't absorbed as easily when they are bogged down by glucose. Too bad eating that salad after a big dessert wasn't as beneficial as I thought. Products high in table sugar and corn syrups create a rapid rise in blood glucose. Blood glucose levels that are always high can cause diseases such as cancer, diabetes, heart disease, hypertension, and yeast infections (Quillin, 2005). Many foods that we eat regularly are already high in glucose such as white rice and bread, so the additional sugar put in just about everything is extra hard on our bodies.

To be called a sugar, the plant has to have 99% of the plant product taken out (the part containing the nutrients), making it highly processed and very rich in nothing but empty calories that spike our blood glucose levels opening the door for disease. The sugars in fruit, called fructose, break down as glucose in our bodies, but have a more positive effect on our blood glucose when eaten as a whole fruit-- fiber included. Dates are a much healthier alternative to sugar because you eat the whole plant. You are going to eat those brownies anyway, right? You might as well eat some sweetened with the whole plant rather than sweetened with a nutrient-less one. Your cells will thank you. And, so will your energy level since it will be sustained.

We teach our kids the importance of brushing our teeth to prevent cavities. Have you ever thought that if something as hard as teeth can be broken down so easily by sugar what other damage can it do to our body parts unseen? Let's start teaching our children to limit the amount of sugar they eat so the cells making their bodies healthy don't get "cavities" either. We unknowingly feed our children junk that we mistake as nutritious. Take a peanut butter and jelly sandwich, for example. Both the bread and the peanut butter likely have sugar and partially hydrogenated oil; the jam has sugar/corn syrup. Put it all together and our children are eating a lot of sugar and trans fat in one item of their lunch. Add in juice, chips, cookies, or yogurt and that is a lot of junk in one meal for their little cells to manage. Luckily, there is usually a jar of jam, in the same aisle of the same store that does not have added sugar; you should be able to also find a natural peanut butter (nothing but peanuts) next to the name brand stuff. There is bread without trans fat and sugar, too, but you have to look really hard in a supermarket. If it's too hard to find a bread without both sugar and trans fat, just pick the one without hydrogenated oils and worry about the sugar later. Cut out what you can. Once you start scrutinizing labels you'll be saddened to know that the marketed healthier whole wheat varieties have more added sugar. It's got to taste good so you'll buy it. We all fall for it. We think it's healthy because it says so, or we just don't pay attention to the sugar content because we don't think to. Also, there is no reason anyone should buy juice with added sweetener (sugar, corn syrup, or the fake stuff). There are plenty of options that taste delicious without added sugar. Sure, you could find a bottle of juice that contains corn syrup for only 99 cents, and the unsweetened varieties can cost around $4, but when you add 1 part juice to 1 part sparkling water flavored with lime you make it last longer and the flavor remains the same. Plus, you can still have something fizzy when you go through soda withdrawals. Paying for cheaper, less healthy items up front will save you money in the short term, but when you suffer from all the diseases we are at risk for, you will be spending more in the long run.

Now with the information I learned about sugar, I had to decide that I wanted to eat to live, not live to eat. At first, the change was easy because I was so upset over my mom's diagnosis and so angry at the sugar manufacturing companies that I wanted nothing to do with the stuff. I actually lost the craving after being away from it for a while and didn't even have any type of dessert for Thanksgiving for the first time ever, but, it slowly crept back in when I gave in to some cake at a birthday party here and something else there. I learned to throw away half of the slice of cake right away to avoid eating too much like I would have in the past. My dad used to tell me, "Better to waste in the trash than to waste in your body." I steered clear of the heavily sweetened products, such as soda. I found other alternatives to satisfy certain cravings, such as making my own hot chocolate with only three ingredients, that is tastier than the packaged stuff (whisk together on low heat until dissolved: 1 cup milk, 1 T cocoa powder, 1 T maple syrup). I started using pure maple syrup for sweetening my oatmeal instead of my former beloved brown sugar. I learned how to like things minimally sweetened, which was a gradual process, but if I can do it, I know you can, too.

Back to my point on how sugar affected me... A year after my first baby was born, I decided I needed caffeine again in order to function at work since dear baby still didn't sleep through the night and I found myself struggling to stay awake in the afternoons. Only this time I knew better than to sweeten my coffee with sugar; however, the thought of drinking unsweetened coffee disgusted me. I just couldn't tolerate coffee without sugar, so I tried black tea. At that time, McDonald's came out with their iced sweet tea, so I asked for half sweetened and half unsweetened until eventually I was able to fade out the sweetened half altogether. I tried an assortment of black teas until I found one I liked unsweetened (Early Grey), and I didn't even mind the taste of some stevia added in once in a while (stevia in coffee is awful so don't even try it). Remember, I came from drinking a super sweet Thai Iced tea almost daily. I told myself the first thing I wanted after I had my baby and was done nursing, was a Thai Iced tea-- but I never had one again, and don't even miss it. The sugar is just not worth it. So, eventually I was back on caffeine just like my grad school days. Only this time, I remained alert, happy, energized. No strange dreams; no more chronic PMS-- no PMS ever. Loud noises were no longer painful. I stopped needing to wrap my knee in the winter. I didn't need naps anymore. It was never the caffeine; it was the sugar all along!

I am not completely sugar free, but use it-- as what I have defined for myself-- "in moderation," so that I still feel good about the health of my cells and my body is not suffering like in the past. I threw away the majority of the recipes I collected over the years, but kept some really great cake recipes that I may make once every couple of years for a celebration, but I might just feel too guilty grabbing for a box of sugar. I pride myself that my oldest son is starting to be conscientious about what he is eating, and, at times, he turns down treats offered to him-- even cupcakes at a birthday party. I do not deprive him of treats, but I control what enters our home. Before he started school, treats included healthier energy bars (in place of candy bars), real-fruit snacks and dark chocolate (in place of candy). When he first started preschool, I saw him during snack time picking out all of the frosted cheerios and putting them back. When his friends asked him why he was doing that, he said they had sugar in them. He didn't do that for long as he saw everyone else happily enjoying them. Unfortunately, schools offer enough junk during the holidays that make me cringe. The influence on others is great. If all of his friends are eating it, then mom must be the weird one. But if mom brings a special treat to school and all of the kids love it, then mom is the cool one and all of his friends, and their parents, can learn about making changes where they can. Since he is informed, and not deprived, I know the seed planted in him will continue to grow.

Transgenic Food (aka Genetically Modified Organism)

GMO. Scientists are manually extracting a trait of some organism(s) and are implanting it into the seeds of soybeans, corn, canola, sugar beets, cotton, alfalfa, Hawaiian papaya, and summer squash to make them disease resistant and/or more efficient to grow (Monsanto.com). It doesn't sound so bad when you hear of vitamin A being inserted into rice for developing countries. Even I used to secretly wish they would find some trait that made plants age slowly and implant them into flowers so we could enjoy cut ones longer—that is, until I started thinking about how the bees that pollinated them would live too long and get super strong just like how they are having trouble with the "super weed." Maybe that super weed got its incessant life from the pollen that got mixed in from the GM crops-- you know the genetically altered crops with the traits that are resistant to herbicides.

GMOs don't sound as good when they are taking from soil a bacteria that is toxic to some bugs and are implanting that toxic trait into our crops, like corn for example. The bugs get sick after first bite and die soon after. They have somehow determined that the bacteria is safe for humans, but there is a great deal of controversy out there. How many humans eat dirt anyway? Remember my rant about PHO? How manually adding hydrogen to a liquid in order to form a solid created trans fat? PHOs were considered to be a healthier alternative for decades, but are now being phased out of our food.

I have three friends that have food allergies severe enough that their bodies are being attacked by the food they eat. It's not my parents' friends that are having trouble with food, it's my friends-- the generations that began ingesting GMOs during childhood, which may or may not be a coincidence. Supporters of GMO say it's harmless to us. (Supposedly cooking in Teflon pans is harmless, too, but it can kill pet birds). What effect does it have on us that we don't see immediately? The effects on us, a larger and more resilient species, may not be noticed until years later and that makes it difficult to pin point the cause. Research supports that food sensitivities are a cause of inflammation, that is, Inflammation in your intestinal barrier lining. So we don't get sick and die like the bugs, yes, that is true. Instead, the inflammation causes us to gain weight which is another epidemic in America: obesity. Add in all the sugary stuff we eat, and guess what? Sugar prevents the good bacteria from doing its job and the result: more inflammation. Once our intestinal barrier is damaged by the food we are sensitive to we may gain weight, acquire diabetes, heart disease, allergies, and other autoimmune diseases (Lanzisera, 2015).

The food that people have most sensitivities to are corn, soy, wheat, and dairy (Lanzisera, 2015). All of those have something to do with GMO except for wheat, so we can't blame GMO for everything. Unless, and I am just throwing this out there, that the sensitivities that may be created within our bodies from the GMOs are exacerbated when mixed with the gluten (the protein found in wheat). It all happens on a level far more advanced than our minds can understand and we may never know. Hence the reason I am avoiding GMO as much as possible since I am far too skeptical when nature didn't intend something to be a certain way as I believe a Perfect Designer originally created perfect food. I look for organic corn and organic soy products because they are not GMO (unless it gets pollinated by accident), but with that being said, only 70% of the product needs to be organic in order to be termed "organic."

Wheat, Dairy, & Allergies

A few years later, just when I figured out how to choose better food, I learned yet another devastating fact about something I was eating. Baby number two was coming along, so I stopped using the three prescribed topical medications for a chronic itchy scalp problem that I had for years. I finally went to get treatment a couple years prior to becoming pregnant again. The problem never did go away, but it was sort of controlled with the medication. I suffered with an itchy scalp all throughout my pregnancy. Once baby was born I had some pounds to lose, so I went on a no-low carb diet. Two weeks later, I realized my scalp problem had vanished. What medications could not permanently fix, my diet was able to. The only thing I cut down on was carbohydrates/calories that I got from wheat and milk. Prior to this, I did not have anything against wheat or dairy. I don't know if it was one or the other or the combination of both. I told my dermatologist about it and she replied, "People have told me that their rash disappeared on a gluten free diet." She never did prescribe me a diet though; it was always meds. Of course, I acknowledge that medications are necessary for many reasons and I am certainly not encouraging anyone to go against any doctor's recommendations. I suggest that while you are being treated with medications you take a serious look at your diet and try cutting out some things. Besides healing my chronic itchy scalp, I had more energy without needing to be caffeinated when I returned back to work on this low carb diet. (If you are curious, I followed Bob Harper's *Skinny Meals*, and lost eight pounds in two weeks.) For the first three months back at work I ate a salad for lunch with a low carb dressing every day. Then, one day, I had to hurriedly grab something for lunch and took a microwavable frozen pasta dinner (yes it had wheat, but I was desperate). This was the first day that I nodded off in the afternoon at work since baby was born. Coincidence? I think not.

Dairy is an issue for many people. Some believe that everyone is lactose intolerant after infancy. People who have an overwhelmed system from food sensitivities have issues with milk proteins looking the same as the gluten proteins (Petersen, 2015). Also, there is evidence to support that there is a strong relationship between type I diabetes and dairy consumption (Petersen, 2015). The sugars in milk may not be so bad for our bodies if overall sugar intake is already low (Ansel, 2015), which is unlikely in an American diet. You can decide that for yourself taking into account what you put milk in-- sugary cereal, oatmeal with brown sugar, overly sweetened coffee, cream in desserts, etc. Might be a good reason to actually define what "in moderation" means more specifically for you.

At the beginning of my healthy food quest, a friend happened to mention to me that he always gets migraines when he eats cheese from a certain store, but never when he eats cheese from Trader Joe's. I thought it was sort of silly since cheese is cheese, right? Later when I got label savvy, I learned that Trader Joe's cheese has fewer preservatives than cheese from other places. It was likely a preservative that triggered my friend's migraines. I found out the hard way, in adulthood, that my migraines were brought on by MSG, which can also be found in some dairy products (such as ultra-pasteurized). Throughout childhood, a couple of times a year, I suffered from excruciatingly painful migraines which included throwing up. My sister and I always got them around the same time which made sense since we ate the same things. We were prescribed pain killers, but were never able to keep them down. At that time, not enough was known about the cause of migraines and certainly there wasn't enough talk about them being linked to food. My mom knew that MSG may not be good for us, so she made sure we ate at Chinese restaurants that did not use MSG and she bought seasonings that were MSG-free. We ate at a Mexican-type fast food restaurant pretty often not knowing that MSG was in all of the food we liked to eat there. I discovered this in adulthood when the nutritional facts and ingredients were available online. It still makes my stomach turn thinking about how I felt when I knew a migraine was coming on: blurry/squiggly vision in one eye or temporary unilateral paralysis of entire body. Then, the massive headache as if a freight train was squishing my brain. Ugh.... I had to lay in bed all day until it worked its way out. It was a cycle of throwing up causing enough relief in order to be able to fall asleep, then waking up again to throw up, etc. Some people can function with chronic migraines, albeit feeling miserable, but able to remain at work. I wouldn't want that lighter version either. Recently, I read a blurb in an article that children who chew gum are getting headaches. I blame the artificial sweeteners. Even though sugar and I don't get along, I would choose it over the fake stuff. My brother-in-law was a diet soda fanatic and suffered from chronic migraines. He finally cut out the diet soda and no longer has migraines. It really was that simple. Recently, my cousin found that her frequent migraines were due to lack of magnesium in her diet since her life was so busy she wasn't able to eat more healthfully. If you suffer from migraines, try taking a good look at your diet while also consulting your doctor. The point is, what we feed our bodies affects every one of us in some way. Let's make changes where we can and minimize or eliminate any sort of suffering!

When I was in college, I kept hearing that if children are displaying bizarre behaviors and/or concentration problems to have them checked out for allergies, including food allergies. One of my friends who started experiencing strange reactions to food had to get a special blood test to find the allergies because it wasn't detected with the other tests. When my son was four years old, he went through this phase (once he started refusing naps) where when he was tired he didn't know how to contain himself; he would bite people for no obvious reason and crawl around on the floor. When he was not tired, I could never imagine him doing those things. What would he be like if he maintained a poor diet on top of that, or if he had a food allergy overlooked? I work with a special education team in an elementary school. My job is to identify and assess children suspected to have delays in communication. During my son's phase, a teacher approached me about a student who was unable to stay in his seat; he wandered around the room or crawled on the floor during class time; he couldn't concentrate on the work. When I met the student, he had dark circles under his eyes; he yawned frequently. For a moment, I panicked wondering if this was the fate of my own son. The student didn't have a communication problem, but he did have interesting behaviors. I thought about my own moodiness and fatigue when I had a high sugar diet, but I slept well. Was this kid just sleep deprived? If the parents weren't ensuring sufficient sleep, were they also unaware of what food may not be nourishing his body? Maybe academic intervention could be faded faster as these issues are explored and that parents are willing to follow through. I am certainly not saying that a child diagnosed with a disorder of some sort may be cured through diet, or that diet may cause the problem. But diet is a good place to start while seeking out the help needed for that child to be successful. I acknowledge that diet may not have much to do with some problems. For fun, I read Melanie Warner's book, *Pandora's Lunchbox*. She explains the evolution of processed food (and you will learn not all of it can be called "food") after her own curiosity about how some of the food she had at home never really rotted, such as a 9-month old tub of guacamole. She ends her book with a story about a family who had a son with behavior problems. He was tested for various things but they never found a solid diagnosis. His mother wanted to try going off of processed food for 10 days and his life was transformed. That family's poor diet only affected one of their children in a severe way. Interesting to note that we are not all affected in similar ways. The cellular health of any individual may be improved through a diet void of processed foods even if the effects aren't immediate.

It's certainly not going to hurt to eat more whole food, when I know how it does hurt to eat processed food. And when you avoid processed food you avoid just about everything mentioned in this book: sugar, trans fat, GMO, wheat, dairy, etc. and your energy goes up and you feel so much better! Who wouldn't want to change? Okay, maybe those people who still insist that the sinful sweets are so hard to resist because they taste so good. Well, check out my recipes to taste and see for yourself that healthy food can be as good. Your biggest food critic will not know they are sugar-free, wheat-free, dairy-free, and soy-free. Then, you can say the change was made easy.

3. CHANGE

"Control me self? How?" –Cookie Monster, *Sesame Street*

Now that you are aware of why we should change what we eat for our own cellular health, we have to learn how to be happy with the changes by finding a satisfying substitute in order to avoid falling back to old habits. Change takes time and we have to force ourselves to make that time. Here's another reason: Not too long ago, a friend and I were comparing our salads at lunch. We both had Chinese chicken salads with different dressings. She used a name brand lite sesame style dressing from the dressing aisle of a supermarket. I told her how I loved the flavor of my dressing from Bob Harper's *Skinny Meals* and it was so easy to make. I named off three out of the four ingredients and she cut me off saying "That is already too complicated for me." It only had four ingredients. It takes me less than one minute to whisk together. Would she have changed her mind if I told her that the dressing she used had at least three different sources of genetically modified ingredients, two identified carcinogens, three mystery ingredients, and two preservatives that we need to study more about? The extra exertion of whisking together four ingredients doesn't seem so effortful anymore. It is easier to change knowing this.

Processed Food Cravings

You can still eat the food you like, just make wiser choices. For example, you don't really have to buy your kids that cereal that contains artificial food coloring (red has been linked to increase hyperactivity), hydrogenated oil (trans fat), soy bean oil (GMO, oxidation), corn flour (GMO), modified corn starch (GMO), corn syrup (GMO) and sugar (likely GMO from sugar beets) when there is a comparable one elsewhere that may have only one of those dreadful ingredients, which is a far better choice. It does mean that you may not be able to do your one stop grocery shop anymore. I know it is an unnerving thought having to go to another place, but if you just go once a month and stock up it is do-able. I started ordering miscellaneous grocery items from *Amazon Prime* to cut down on trips to different stores.

Many stores have healthier processed food items now. Start comparing ingredient labels and choose the lesser evil until you have a plan to cut out the processed food item altogether or find a better substitute. I replaced my *Hot Cheetos* addiction to spicy veggie chips, which seem to be a more cell friendly product. I shop mostly at Trader Joe's because they are affordable and have improved processed food substitutes, such as crackers, cereals, chips, energy-type bars, etc. Unfortunately, most of their healthier readymade food contains soy oil, which is a problem if you are avoiding GMO, and increased risk of cell oxidation. The change can be gradual, so give yourself time to adjust. Once you get used to a change, then upgrade again later when you are ready, such as considering making stuff yourself or buying the more expensive substitute at a health food store. Make sure you are still checking labels even if you shop at a health food store because PHOs still sneak in and the GMOs and oils that oxidize easily are everywhere.

Leave the drive thru for emergencies when you really don't have the time rather than stop a few times during the week as regular routine. When you stop to think about all of the MSG, unknown preservatives, artificial sweeteners, sugar, and trans fat and GMOs you will likely be ingesting in just about every bite, making dinner doesn't feel as daunting of a task. Start planning ahead and change your routine a little at a time. Pick just one day of the week to change, and add from there when you have that one day down.

Really for me it came down to opening a bag of chips was way easier than chopping up something healthy. So I encourage you to cut up the veggies as soon as you bring them home or right before you go to bed (it only takes about 10 minutes) and bag them into easy to grab snack packs. It feels so good knowing that you are eating a healthy option in place of an empty calorie version that doesn't just add fat to your body but breaks down your white blood cells. The best part is those veggies are essentially calorie free and they fill you up while taking away the need to munch.

I've gotten into bad habits by needing to snack on things when sitting at the computer. It's like Pavlov's bell rings as soon as I sit down to work on documents. So, I replaced the munchie stuff with a bowl of berries, and in the afternoon if I need something sweet I pull out a piece of dark chocolate instead of cookies. Write a list of all things you eat during the day for a week and decide on what to tackle first once you realize how frequently you eat it, and then replace it.

During one of my mom's chemotherapy infusions, I saw a volunteer pushing a hospitality cart full of, unbeknownst to that person, and likely the administration, snacks with trans fat and/or sugar for the cancer patients and families. My mom took a snack and I scrunched up my nose. When it's so readily available I understand that it's hard to pass up. That is why I started to carry snacks in my purse and in my car (e.g., nuts, healthy snack bars), so that when I'm starving on my way home from work I don't stop at Mc Donald's to get some fries (fried in an easily oxidized oil). Later on, my mom decided to drastically change her diet. She wanted to reduce her sugar intake, and when she announced she was going vegan and soy free my sister rolled her eyes. Those rolled eyes were all too familiar to me, but once a seed is planted it's bound to sprout. It's been about five years since my mom's diagnosis of stage IV cancer, and she is stronger than ever. I'm sure her positive dietary changes have a lot to do with it (and maybe also being a grandma).

I want to mention that there are some cases where people, who need to drink meal replacements, such as Ensure or Pediasure, follow the advice of their doctors even though these drinks are full of sugar and GMO ingredients because it is likely better than not getting enough nutrition at all. We don't know that they have a negative effect for short term use but that they do have a positive effect for a person who needs them. My prayer is that companies manufacturing meal replacements become sensitive to what is actually in the drinks and make positive changes-- especially when immunosuppressed people are the ones drinking it.

Using Oil

- Unrefined Coconut Oil- this oil withstands heat much better than other oils before oxidizing so try the switch for frying. It brings about a slight coconut flavor though, so it doesn't go with everything, like fried eggs. It adds a great flavor to fried organic corn tortillas for tacos; it's great for French Toast, and even gives popcorn a wonderful flavor. I substitute coconut oil in all baked goods that call for canola or other vegetable oil. So far, Trader Joe's has the best price for this. It's currently $5.99 for 16oz. I've seen it in a supermarket as high as $10.49 for 14 oz! Coconut oil is solid at room temperature, so don't be alarmed if it's melted during the summer months.
- Refined Coconut Oil- this oil does not have any coconut flavor; however, all refined oils are heated at a high heat (which causes oxidation), deodorized and bleached by some process to remove impurities, and typically chemicals are added in. Then, when we heat it again at home we cause more oxidation. Coconut oil withstands higher temperatures better than others, but it still breaks down. It's best to avoid all refined oils. Though I suppose roasting your own potatoes in refined coconut oil is better than what you would get on your French fries going to a drive thru.
- Ghee- is a clarified butter product that can withstand hotter temperatures better. Try it with fried eggs.

- Olive Oil- try to stop using this to cook with. What made us think we need to use oil to sauté with in the first place? Use a little water or broth and you won't miss the difference, especially for soups. Olive oil is considered to be a heart healthy oil, except for when it's heated. This oil is best used in salad dressings, dips, and in pastas after cooking. Most olive oils come in darker bottles, which aid in preventing oxidation. The best type is *expeller pressed*, which means it was processed in the dark to limit any oxidation caused from light.
- Vegetable, soybean, corn, and canola oil- I don't recommend using these oils since they easily oxidize and are likely genetically modified. You will be getting this type of oil when you eat out, so don't use it at home.

Replacing Sugar

Around the same time when my mom was being treated with chemotherapy, my sister started to look more into nutrition herself and lost 20 pounds, and her high blood pressure problem was resolved. She started to find healthy food bloggers on the internet and was interested in many of the dessert make-overs. I started experimenting on my own after I came upon a pamphlet on diabetes that included recipes using dates. Dates are a whole plant product, which makes for a more positive effect on blood cholesterol and glucose in our bodies. I thought about how we only bought those coconut date rolls during dried fruit sales at fundraisers during elementary school. It wasn't anything I ever craved. I fell in love with dates when my sister made a *Sugar Free Chocolate Chip Bean Cake Cookie* sweetened with dates from thediva-dish.com. In my recipe section, you will find whole dates as the sweetener for the majority of the recipes. If you don't like dates, you will still enjoy these recipes, according to two of my tasters that had an aversion to dates. Please keep in mind that these recipes are not for losing weight. They are just as rich and satisfying as what you would normally want in a dessert, so they are not calorie friendly. Dates are high in glucose (although absorbed better in the bloodstream than table sugar), so these recipes are not recommended to consume in excess even though they are nutritionally dense. If you have diabetes, you still have to use sparingly and always keep your doctor informed about what you are eating.

- Dates - For every ½ cup of sugar substitute 10 dates. I prefer to use Medjool dates because they are sweeter and softer to process. If you use another brand of dates, you may need to double the amount. I've substituted 2 cups of sugar in a cake with 40 dates. Yes, that's a lot of dates when they are more expensive than sugar, but you don't bake a cake every day. You could also do half sugar and half dates to ease your way into this. I buy whole dates and just split them in half to pit, and toss in the food processor. Overall, I find that I'm not spending any more at the market because I'm no longer buying the processed junk food that was a waste of money. That's a lot of cellular destruction you save, too, you know! So far I have found that Trader Joe's gives you the most dates for the least amount of money.
- Honey and Maple syrup- At first, I started substituting sugar with honey and maple syrup the most, but they are high in glucose so you still have to eventually use sparingly. A tablespoon of sugar is completely nutrient-less whereas a tablespoon of honey and maple syrup have minerals, vitamins, and antioxidants. Once honey is pasteurized, however, it loses a lot of nutrients.
- Agave Nectar and Stevia- Agave nectar has a low glycemic index, but still a highly processed product, so the amount of goodness it does to our bodies is unknown, if any. Stevia tasted terrible in coffee, but tolerable in tea. Stevia is helpful for regulating blood glucose and it's not artificial (unless a specific brand adds things to it).
- Sugar- remember in order to be called a sugar, 99% of the plant product is stripped away leaving us with a dangerously

sweet and nutrient-less product. Try to use sugar as sparingly as possible. Save it for a special occasion, not for daily indulgence. Identify where you consume this the heaviest, and then start cutting back either by substituting or limiting. If you can't cut it out of coffee, for example, (remember it was hard for me, too, but with persistence and motivation you can learn to enjoy unsweetened lattes) then make that your only source of sugar and totally eliminate it elsewhere. So don't get that pastry along with your sweetened beverage. You have to pick and choose here-- or you can just bake your own replacements from my recipe section.

Substituting Candy Bars

Avoid the candy aisles! Go far out of your way if you have to in a store. That was how I cut out my hard candy problem when I was in my late teens. I got a cavity, so decided it wasn't worth it, but I had to not even look at candy. I used to buy *Gobstoppers* or *Nerds* almost every time I stopped at a gas station as a teenager. It was especially difficult at Target during Halloween season, so I made the decision that sugar in that form was just not an option and I had to avoid the temptation. Years after I recovered from my candy vice, and discovered trans fat, I stared long and hard at all of that sugary garbage and had the urge to buy every one of those hundreds of bags in order to throw them away (especially those chocolate log-like candies), but I knew that wouldn't solve the problem. I just didn't want anyone to waste their cells away. Put the money aside that you would have spent on candy and buy something else more important.

If chocolate is your weakness, then start by gradually going darker and darker. When I was a kid it only took tasting dark chocolate one time to know that it wasn't sweet enough. Now, I buy minimum of 72% cocoa and make sure there is no soy product because it will likely be GMO. It's dark enough when sugar isn't the first ingredient. After familiarizing yourself with your supermarket's chocolate bar section, you should be able to find at least one good quality brand that does not add soy.

When trying to cut down on candy bar consumption, check out my chocolate almond, and peanut butter bites recipes (p. 62-64) for popular candy bar cravings, so that you are satisfied without giving in to the trans fat and sugar when it comes to candy bars. Pop one or two of these bites in your mouth when you are sleepy in the afternoon and your energy won't tank. You can also start trying Clif Bars (the kid's *Zbar* have better ingredients) or LaraBars for replacing candy bars. Dark chocolate is really good with cashews or almonds and makes a great afternoon snack. Fruit helps curb sweet cravings, especially apples. Apples are way more appealing when they are sliced and/or peeled. I dislike the flavor combinations of chocolate and cinnamon, so when I crave something chocolaty and sweet, I eat an apple or a peach with cinnamon and then I don't feel like anything with chocolate after that.

Breakfast

At least America has it right that sugar should be eaten for breakfast. Just not in everything! I've included breakfast make-overs in my recipes since we do dessert for breakfast the majority of the time when we eat muffins, waffles, pastries, and even packaged oatmeal. At least you will feel good about what you are rushing out of the door with.

- Sweeten oatmeal with as little maple syrup as possible. Nix the brown sugar. People are misled that brown sugar is somehow healthier because it's "brown." It's the same as white sugar just flavored with molasses. I used to eat it by the spoonful when I needed something sweet. I don't miss it at all anymore because maple syrup has a similar flavor.
- Craving a donut? Try adding cinnamon and freshly ground nutmeg to your oatmeal. It tastes like a plain donut.
- Sick of your oatmeal? Try cooking up steel cut oats. The flavor is greatly enhanced when compared to rolled oats. It takes longer to cook, so when you wake up boil some water, then

while you are getting ready put in the steel cut oats and let simmer coming back to stir every once in a while. Set a timer so you don't forget. My favorite oatmeal is made with peanut butter, maple syrup, pecans with unsweetened almond milk with a sliced banana.

- Dying for a scone at your favorite coffee shop? My mouth used to salivate at the sight of Starbucks' maple oat scones, but as soon as I got into the car with my unsweetened latte, the craving was gone. Out of sight out of mind. I do have a maple oat biscuit recipe that makes a good substitute (p. 46).
- Always buy pure maple syrup to have on hand. You have to pay more for it, but it's worth the expense and you'll use it more sparingly. If you enjoy going to pancake houses once in a while, then bring a little pure maple syrup with you to add on a little more nutrients to that nutrient-less pancake.
- If you normally have a cake-like breakfast every day, then start by reducing to every other day to once a week, etc.

Using Milk

My recipes are dairy free, but not because I am encouraging a vegan diet. I want these recipes to suit any lifestyle. There is some controversy about whether we should be drinking animal milk, but if you drink milk, I recommend that you buy organic cow's milk since those cows likely have a better diet. Some non-dairy milk selections can have an added ingredient that has raised some concern called *carrageenan,* but there is always a brand that doesn't have it added. Many of the first things people substitute for cow's milk is soy milk. If you grab soy milk you're likely getting one with added sugar. Unsweetened soy milk is not that great as a drink on its own, so the sweetened variety makes it taste more like milk, but then you just added more sugar into your diet. You want to make sure it's organic if you want to avoid the GMO stuff. I always have unsweetened organic soy milk on hand to use in savory dishes, which is great for those who are lactose intolerant. You won't be able to tell the difference in creamy gravies, and even chicken pot pie, for example.

Replacing Soda

Many people are not willing to give up soda whether it is diet or fully loaded. It is quite addictive. Start by ordering a medium instead of a large; then a small instead of a medium; pour half of the can down the drain immediately after you open it. After I weaned myself off of soda, I still craved a Coke every once in a while, so I just took a couple of sips to satisfy my cravings, but that requires that you are willing and ready to commit to immediately throwing it out so you don't have too much. Do the same with whatever food vices you have. Just throw out half of it immediately (like the slice of cake at a birthday party). If you deprive yourself too much for too long you could end up overdoing it in one sitting. Just don't have it at home, and only have it when you eat out (but be careful of free refills), then fade it out more over time.

For some reason a lot of people don't like water probably because it's flavorless and we have corrupted our palates with far too many sugary drinks. Start by adding in lemon, lime, mint, cucumber, or even pineapple to give it some flavor. Try sparkling water and replace soda with 1 part sparkling lime water with 1 part 100% juice and have a healthier soda.

Coffee

Learn to like it black. Yes, that is possible. I loved sugar so much, when my friend gave me a ¼ tray of baklava I ate it all in one day. Daily, I had to have sweet drinks whether it was soda, Thai Iced Tea (that I had so often I learned how to make myself) or a Starbucks *Frappucino* (which I also learned how to make similarly). Before I knew about the devastating effects of sugar on my body, I would have never wanted to go anywhere near black coffee. When I decided that sugar was just not an option, I had to learn how to like things less sweetened- which was a long and gradual process, but, I did it. And so can you! I have had so much success (however, still do cave maybe once a month rather than every day) that now when I eat a real dessert it tastes far too sweet. I wanted so badly to like unsweetened coffee so I started adding in more milk, which made it tolerable. Eventually, I learned to love unsweetened lattes because the milk adds a subtle sweetness that was far better than black. Then, I learned about coffee beans when Starbucks posted the notification that *acrylamide* is a known carcinogen. Acrylamide occurs naturally when just about anything is roasted and browned (e.g., baked potatoes, cookies, coffee beans). So no wonder certain coffees are revoltingly bitter when not doctored up with a lot of cream and sugar-- they are burned beans. I'd like to not eat or drink anything that may be cancerous since I know I'm bombarded with environmental carcinogens all day that are not in my immediate control. So, for that reason I looked for light roasts, and they tasted amazing black, but you just can't go for the cheap stuff here. High quality makes all of the difference. Imagine sipping a dark roast *black* with the utterly bitter aftertaste compared to a high-end light roast that has a surprisingly caramel-like aftertaste. What an incredible difference. If you still can't go black you could at least go from eight packets of sugar to two when drinking the lighter roasts. If you have a bean roaster in your community I highly encourage you to check out their light roasts. Other great alternatives for bitter-less flavor are Gevalia and Farmer Brothers brands. I used to guzzle down the sweetened coffee drinks within 5 minutes, but now I savor the flavor of the coffee and enjoy it longer.

<u>Desserts in General</u>

Let's say I really want a pastry. All I have to do is tell myself that 1) I will not eat trans fat because it causes my cellular health to suffer and can clog my arteries even though it's unsaturated fat; 2) the wheat and/or dairy will flare up my scalp dermatitis; 3) there are genetically modified ingredients in it and I don't feel comfortable not knowing what they may do to me; 4) the sugar is going to make me want more and then I will suffer more and chance having joint pain, moodiness, or even worse lower my immunity. That pastry just totally lost its appeal. When you tell yourself that a certain food is just not an option you learn how to get something healthier in its place and you eventually lose the cravings. I could care less about packaged cookies now, when before I could eat a whole box at once. Even a friend tried to pressure me into eating one and I had zero desire. I would much rather spend my calories eating something that packs a lot of nutrients per bite that is not sickening sweet, but clean and guilt free.

You will lose the sugary craving much easier the longer you are away from it. If you have to give in to something, then just make sure it doesn't have trans fat along with the sugar. If you love something that contains both, you will be successful in finding another alternative that is better for your body by shopping around and familiarizing yourself with the ingredient labels.

 When you eat a dessert, you are likely eating all of the things mentioned above (sugar, trans fat, wheat, dairy, and transgenic food) that have a negative effect on our bodies. My recipes were created to taste just like the real desserts we all know and love. Go ahead and feel good eating dessert-- even for breakfast!

4. RECIPES

Special Equipment: You will need a food processor in order to process the dates. If you don't already have one, it is worth the small investment because you can make your own dips, pesto, hummus, and salsas so easily-- without all of the bad oils. I recommend at least a 9-cup food processor. I use a blender, an ice cream maker, and a waffle maker for a couple of the recipes as well.

Oats: If you have a gluten allergy then you will want to buy gluten free (GF) oats. Typically, oats are processed on the same equipment as wheat, so the gluten may get mixed in. GF oats are milled on designated equipment. I buy the oats in bulk rather than buying oat flour because I save money that way. I am going to dirty up my food processor with the dates anyway, so processing the oats first is quick and easy. You can use oat flour that is already made using the same measurements.

Dates: see page 28 for more information regarding dates.

Milk: I typically have unsweetened almond milk on hand, but you can use whatever type of unsweetened milk you enjoy for these recipes.

Flax seed: I use ground flax seed as the egg substitute, but if you have to avoid eating flax seed (e.g., it can interfere with some medications), then you can use chia seed: 1 T chia seeds in 2 T water; set aside until gelled, then mix in as you would the flax seed according to the recipe.

Dark Chocolate Chips: The one exception to my sugar free baking is using dark chocolate chips in certain recipes. I use Enjoy Life brand found at health food markets. The recipes that include dark chocolate chips are still healthier than the regular desserts out there. Most chocolate chips have a soy product in them, but if you are new to reading labels then worry about that later.

Some people have mistakenly believed that these recipes are labor intensive. Far from the truth. It doesn't take any longer than a regular recipe. The best part is that the majority of these recipes are made in one bowl (the food processor bowl), which makes clean up easy!

Most everything freezes nicely and makes great food gifts!

Banana Nut Muffins

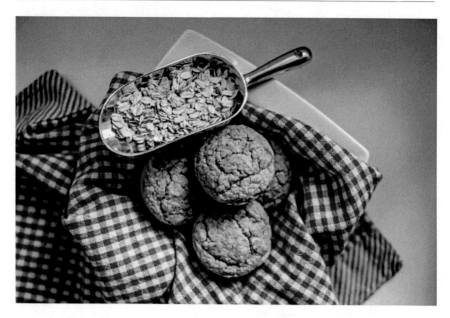

Lightly sweetened with dates, these muffins make a guilt free breakfast, and a fun way to eat oatmeal in the mornings.

- 2 cups rolled oats
- 6 Medjool dates, pitted, halved
- 1 T baking powder
- 1 T ground flax seed
- ½ tsp salt
- 1 cup unsweetened almond milk
- 1 tsp vanilla extract
- 3/4 cup mashed overripe banana
- 1/3 cup coconut oil, melted (plus more for greasing the muffin tin)
- 1/2 cup chopped walnuts, optional

In a food processor, grind oats into flour. Add the dates. Pulse a few times to break them up, and then grind until the mixture is sandy. Add in the baking powder, flax seed, and salt. Add the vanilla to the almond milk. With the food processor on, slowly pour in the milk mixture. Add the mashed banana and pulse to combine. With the food processor on, slowly pour in the oil. Add the walnuts pulsing a few times to mix them in. Scoop the batter into a greased muffin tin (grease by dipping a napkin in melted coconut oil and smear around tin). If the mixture is too runny, let it sit for a few minutes before scooping into the muffin tin.

Bake at 400°F for about 12-15 minutes. Makes 8 regular sized muffins or about 20 mini muffins.

Spice Muffins

Wonderful to have during the holidays, or anytime, really.

- 2 cups rolled oats
- 8 Medjool dates, pitted, halved
- 1 T ground flax
- 1 T baking powder
- 1 tsp ground cinnamon
- ½ tsp ground ginger
- ½ tsp ground allspice
- Pinch ground cloves
- Pinch ground nutmeg
- 1 cup unsweetened almond milk
- 1 tsp vanilla extract
- 1/3 cup coconut oil, melted (plus more for greasing the muffin tin)

In a food processor, grind oats into flour. Add the dates. Pulse a few times to break them up, and then grind until the mixture is sandy. Add in the baking powder, flax seed, and spices. Add the vanilla to the almond milk. With the food processor on, slowly pour in the milk mixture. Add the coconut oil and pulse to combine. Scoop batter into a greased muffin tin (grease by dipping a napkin in melted coconut oil and smear around tin).

Bake at 400°F for about 12 minutes or until a toothpick inserted in the center comes out clean. Makes about 8 regular-sized or 20 mini muffins.

Lemon Poppy Seed Muffins

Lemon lovers will be impressed!

- 2 cups rolled oats
- 12 Medjool dates, pitted, halved
- 1 T baking powder
- 1 T ground flax
- 1 cup unsweetened almond milk
- 2 T lemon zest (about 4 lemons)
- ¼ cup poppy seeds, optional
- 1/3 cup coconut oil, melted (plus more for greasing the muffin tin)

In a food processor, grind oats into flour. Add the dates. Pulse a few times to break them up, and then grind until the mixture is sandy. Add in the baking powder, and flax seed; pulse to combine. Pour in the almond milk; pulse to combine. Add the lemon zest and poppy seeds; pulse to combine. Pour in the coconut oil with the machine on just until incorporated in the batter. Spoon into greased muffin tin (grease by dipping a napkin in melted coconut oil and smear around tin).

Bake at 400°F for about 12 minutes. Makes about 8 regular sized muffins or 20 mini muffins.

Blueberry Zucchini Muffins

Nice way to sneak in veggies! No anti-vegetable child will know they have zucchini in them if you just call them blueberry muffins.

- 2 cups rolled oats
- 10 Medjool dates, pitted, halved
- 1 tsp baking soda
- 1 tsp cinnamon
- ½ tsp salt
- ½ tsp baking powder
- 3 T ground flax seed
- 1 tsp pure vanilla extract
- ¾ cup coconut oil, melted
- 2 cups shredded zucchini
- 1 cup blueberries (fresh or frozen)

In a food processor, grind oats into flour. Add the dates. Pulse a few times to break them up, and then grind until the mixture is sandy. Pulse in the baking soda, cinnamon, salt, baking powder, flax seed. Pulse in the vanilla. With the machine running, add the coconut oil until combined. Add the zucchini giving quick pulses to mix in, and then add the blueberries giving quick pulses just to mix in. Spoon into a greased muffin tin (grease by dipping a napkin in melted coconut oil and smear around tin).

Bake at 350°F for about 15 minutes. Makes approximately 10 regular sized muffins or 24 mini muffins.

Chocolate Chip Muffins

Yes, chocolate for breakfast in a healthy way!

- 2 cups rolled oats
- 10 Medjool dates, pitted, halved
- 1 T baking powder
- 1 T ground flax seed
- 1 cup unsweetened almond milk
- 1 tsp vanilla extract
- 1/3 cup coconut oil, melted (plus more for greasing the muffin tin)
- ½ cup mini dark chocolate chips

In a food processor, grind oats into flour. Add the dates. Pulse a few times to break them up, and then grind until the mixture is sandy. Add in the baking powder, and flax seed; pulse to combine. Pour in the almond milk with the vanilla extract; pulse to combine. With the machine running, pour in the coconut oil. Add in the chocolate chips and pulse a few times to combine. Spoon into a greased muffin tin (grease by dipping a napkin in melted coconut oil and smear around tin).

Bake in 400°F for about 12 minutes. Makes about 8 regular sized muffins, or 20 mini muffins.

Chocolate Waffles

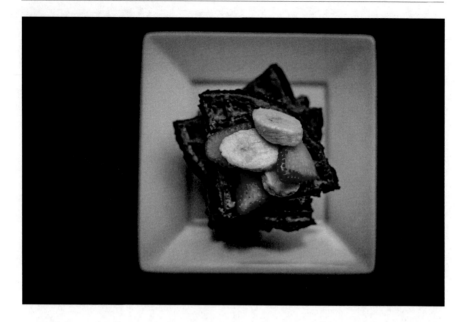

I usually make these waffles without the dates because I like to drizzle maple syrup over them, so they don't need any extra sweetener. These are great topped with banana and strawberry slices, or any frozen berries, warmed. Definitely a great waffle to impress company with at breakfast. Make it even fancier by adding a scant amount of dark chocolate chips as a topping. Go ahead, put on the real whipped cream if you want, since it's healthier than what you would buy on a brunch menu anyway.

- 1 ½ cups rolled oats
- 10 Medjool dates, pitted, halved, optional
- 2 T ground flax seed
- ½ cup cocoa powder
- 2 tsp baking powder
- 2 cups unsweetened almond milk
- 1 ½ tsp vanilla extract
- 4 T coconut oil, melted

In a food processor, grind oats into flour. Add the dates, if using. Pulse a few times to break them up, and then grind until the mixture is sandy. Mix in the flax seed, cocoa powder, and baking powder. Add in the almond milk with the vanilla; pulse to combine. Add the coconut oil to combine. If the batter is too thin, let it sit a few minutes. Follow directions to your waffle iron.

Makes about 4 waffles.

Grab 'N Go Waffles

No need for maple syrup. Make a big batch and freeze them. Pop them in the toaster for rushed mornings and go. Your kids will love them as much as you will.

- 2 cups rolled oats
- 5 Medjool dates, pitted, halved
- 3 tsp baking powder
- 2 T ground flax seed
- 1 tsp freshly ground nutmeg
- 1 tsp vanilla extract
- 1 ½ cups unsweetened almond milk
- 4 T coconut oil, melted

In a food processor, grind oats into flour. Add the dates. Pulse a few times to break them up, and then grind until the mixture is sandy. Add in the baking powder, flax seed, and nutmeg. Combine the vanilla with the almond milk. While the food processor is running, add the milk mixture. Then pour in the coconut oil. Follow directions to your waffle iron. The batter will be runny at first, but will thicken up.

Makes about 4 large waffles.

Maple Oat Biscuits with Glaze

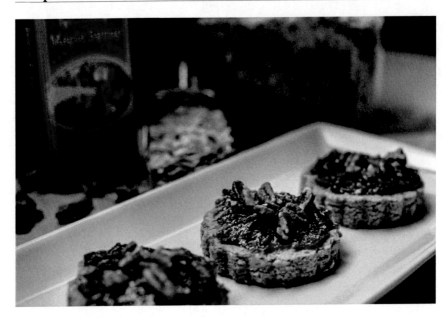

These should replace your desire for that breakfast pastry. You can find coconut and almond flours at Trader Joe's, a health food store, or Amazon.com.

- 1 cup rolled oats
- 10 Medjool dates, pitted, halved
- ½ cup coconut flour
- ½ cup almond meal/flour
- 1 T baking powder
- Generous pinch of salt
- 2 T ground flax seed
- 2 T coconut oil, melted
- 1 tsp vanilla extract
- ¼- ½ cup unsweetened almond milk, if necessary.

In a food processor, grind the oats into a flour; add the dates. Pulse a few times to break them up. Then add the remainder of the dry ingredients; pulse until the dough is a sandy texture. Add the vanilla extract and coconut oil, pulse until combined. If the dough is too dry add ¼ cup almond milk and more if necessary up to ½ cup. Dump the dough out on a board and shape into a disk about an inch thick. Cut into wedges like a pie, or cut out shapes. Place onto a Silpat or greased cookie sheet.

Bake at 350°F for about 15 minutes. When cooled, add the glaze. Makes about 6 biscuits.

Glaze:

- 4 Medjool dates, pitted, halved
- ¼ cup maple syrup
- ¼ tsp vanilla extract
- 2-4 T unsweetened almond milk
- ¼ cup pecan pieces for sprinkling on the top

Process altogether starting with 2 T milk. If it needs to be thinner add more up to 4 tablespoons. Spoon onto the cooled biscuits, top with pecan pieces.

Cinnamon Roll Spread

If you can't get a cinnamon roll out of your mind, then eat this with toast and you should be satisfied.

- 6 Medjool dates, pitted, halved
- 1 tsp ground cinnamon
- Walnut pieces

Process the dates with the cinnamon until the mixture gathers into a ball. Spread on toast; sprinkle some walnut pieces over the toast. Try to use within a day to avoid refrigeration because it will become too hard to spread.

Serves approximately 4.

Blueberry Jam

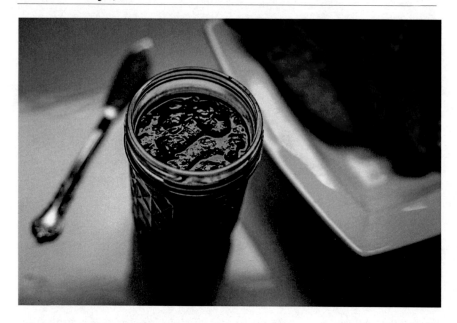

If you like jam on the tart side, which I do, you will need to add a sprinkle of chia seed to thicken it up. If you prefer the sweeter side, then the dates will thicken it up, and it couldn't be easier to make with just two ingredients.

- 6 oz box of fresh or frozen blueberries
- 3-6 Medjool dates, pitted, halved
- 1 tsp chia seed, if using only 3 dates

Cook blueberries on low heat, covered, until bubbly. Process the blueberries with the dates, but cover the machine with a towel to avoid hot splatter. If using chia seed, pour blueberry mixture into a bowl and mix in the chia seeds using a whisk. It will thicken in a few minutes. Store in the refrigerator.

Makes about 6 oz.

Pumpkin Butter

Nothing welcomes autumn like pumpkin butter. It's especially comforting to know there isn't any sugar in it. I make my own pumpkin spice because I have all of the spices on hand. I use approximately ½ tsp cinnamon, pinch of ground ginger, sprinkle of cloves, ground allspice, and freshly ground nutmeg.

- 10 Medjool dates, pitted, halved
- 1 cup pumpkin puree (about 1/2 of a can)
- ¼ tsp pure vanilla extract
- ½ tsp pumpkin spice

In a food processor, process the dates by themselves until they are like a puree. Add the remaining ingredients using quick pulses until it is all combined and the date pieces are hardly noticeable. You will need to stop and scrape down the sides of the bowl a few times. Spread on toast. Keep in the refrigerator for up to one week.

Makes about one cup.

Peach Cobbler

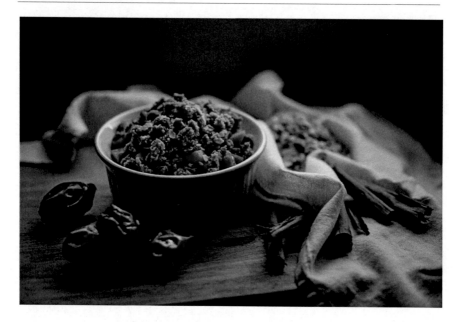

This one is definitely a favorite among my friends. If peaches are out of season, make apple cobbler instead. Peel and slice one apple per serving and steam on top of the stove to help soften them. Sprinkle in some cinnamon and add about a tablespoon of maple syrup along with the apples.

- 2/3 cup rolled oats, divided
- 6 Medjool dates, pitted, halved
- 1 tsp ground flax seed
- 1/4 tsp baking powder
- 1/4 tsp ground cinnamon
- 1/4 tsp vanilla extract
- ¼ cup coconut oil, melted
- 4 large, ripe peaches (about one peach per serving)

In a food processor, grind 1/3 cup of the rolled oats. Add the dates until sandy. Pulse in the flax seed, baking powder, and cinnamon just to combine. While processor is running, add the vanilla and coconut oil until combined. Pulse in the remaining 1/3 cup oats, but keep them mostly whole. Set aside (or refrigerate until ready to use within a couple of days). Peel and chop the peaches. Toss in some additional cinnamon to lightly coat the peaches. Stuff the peaches into three-four ramekins and pack on the topping.

Bake at 350°F for about 15 minutes. Serves 4.

Hot Cocoa

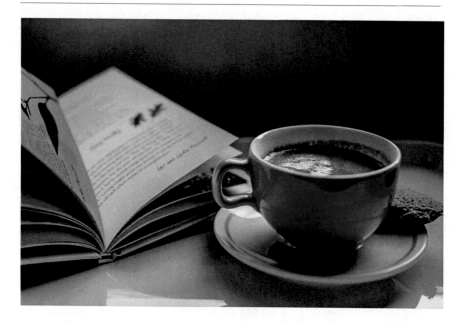

This is a healthier alternative to all the packaged hot chocolates out there.

- 2 cups unsweetened almond milk
- 2 T cocoa powder
- 3 T pure maple syrup
- 1 tsp coconut cream, optional

In a small sauce pan over medium heat, whisk together all ingredients until the cocoa powder dissolves and is warmed. If you have any coconut cream left over from a recipe that doesn't use a whole can (like the brown rice pudding), then try it in this hot cocoa.

Makes 2 servings.

Grandma Jean's Persimmon Cookies

My Grandma's persimmon cookies were my childhood favorite and I still love to bake them when persimmons are in season-- only I have changed a few things, like substituting the butter, flour, and sugar with healthier ingredients. Use the raindrop-shaped persimmons.

- 3 cups rolled oats
- 20 Medjool dates, pitted, halved
- ½ tsp salt
- ½ tsp ground nutmeg
- 1 tsp cinnamon
- 1 tsp baking soda
- 1 tsp baking powder
- 1 T ground flax seed
- 1 tsp vanilla extract
- 1 cup persimmon puree (about three very ripe rain-drop persimmons)
- 1 tsp lemon juice
- 2 T orange juice
- ¼ cup coconut oil, melted
- ¾ cup chopped walnuts

In a food processor, grind the oats into a flour; add the dates half at a time until the mixture is a course sand. Add remaining dry ingredients, pulse to combine. Add the vanilla, persimmon puree, lemon, and orange juices. Pulse a few times to combine. Add the coconut oil and pulse until combined. Add the chopped walnuts, and pulse a few times to incorporate in the dough. Drop by spoonfuls on a Silpat or greased cookie sheet.

Bake at 375°F for 12 minutes. Makes about 4 dozen.

PB&J Cookies

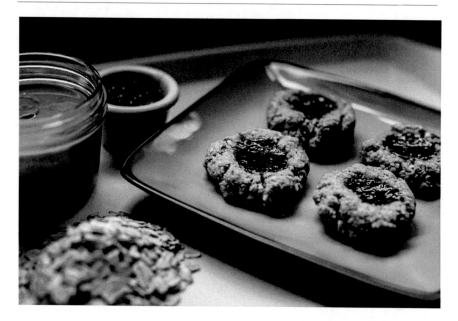

These are fun cookies that remind me of those Smucker's *Uncrustables*, but a healthier version.

- 2 cups rolled oats
- 7 Medjool dates, pitted, halved
- 2 tsp baking powder
- 1 tsp salt
- 1 T ground flax seed
- 1 cup unsweetened almond milk
- 1 tsp vanilla extract
- ¾ cup peanut butter (nothing added but peanuts)
- Strawberry or grape jelly, no sweetener added

In a food processor, grind the oats into flour; pulse in the dates, then turn machine on until sandy. Mix in the baking powder, salt, flax seed. Combine the vanilla extract with the almond milk and pour into the batter with the machine running. Add the peanut butter and pulse in until totally combined. Drop by spoonfuls onto a Silpat or greased cookie sheet. Push the centers of the cookies down with a spoon, to form a well, and fill with jelly.

Bake at 350°F for about 14 minutes. Makes about 12 cookies.

Grain-free Coconut Cookies

I am more of a chocolate person myself, but these are surprisingly delicious. You can find coconut flour at Trader Joe's, a health food store, or Amazon.com.

- 1/4 cup coconut flour
- 12 Medjool dates, pitted, halved
- 1 T ground flax seed
- ½ tsp vanilla extract
- 1 cup unsweetened shredded coconut
- ¼ cup coconut oil, melted

In a food processor, pulse the first five ingredients together until crumbly. Add the oil at the end until incorporated. Drop by rounded spoonfuls on a Silpat or greased cookie sheet.

Bake at 350°F for about 10 minutes. Makes one dozen.

Grain-free Chocolate Heart Cookies

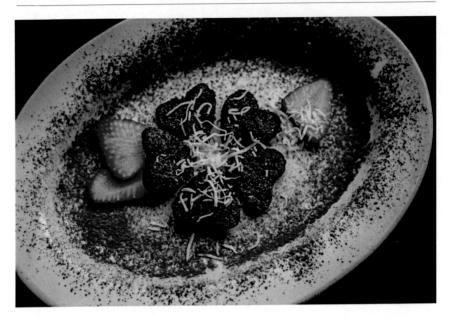

These taste like the chocolate almond bites, but in the form of a cookie for those of you who would rather have a cookie. This recipe also makes great "dirt" for those kids food projects (but leave out the baking soda).

- 12 Medjool dates, pitted, halved
- ½ cup almond flour
- ¼ cup cocoa powder
- ½ tsp baking soda
- 1 tsp pure vanilla extract
- ½ cup unsweetened, shredded coconut
- ¼ cup dark chocolate chips
- 1 T coconut oil, melted

Process the first 6 ingredients until the mixture is like a fine sand. Add the remaining ingredients and keep the machine running until the mixture starts to create small clumps meaning that when it's pressed together it will hold its shape. Place a cookie cutter shape on a cutting board and push down some of the dough into the cookie cutter no more than ½ inch thick. Remove the cookie cutter and repeat with the remaining dough. Transfer the shapes onto a greased cookie sheet or Silpat.

Bake at 350°F for no more than 6 minutes. Makes about 16 cookies.

Cinnamon Raisin Cookies

The new oatmeal-raisin cookie.

- 1 ¼ cup rolled oats
- 1 ½ cup almond meal
- 20 Medjool dates, pitted, halved
- 2 T ground flax seed
- 2 tsp baking powder
- 2 tsp ground cinnamon
- ½ tsp salt
- ½ cup unsweetened almond milk
- ½ cup coconut oil, melted
- ½ cup raisins

In a food processor, pulse the oats into a flour; pulse in the almond meal, dates, flax seed, baking powder, cinnamon, salt until sandy. Drizzle in the almond milk with the machine on. Then drizzle in the coconut oil with the machine running. Add the raisins and give a few quick pulses to mix in. Place rounded spoonfuls on a cookie tray, preferably on a Silpat, about one inch apart.

Bake at 350°F for about 12 minutes. Makes approximately three dozen.

Chocolate Covered Cookie Dough Balls (on cover)

A raw cookie dough you can eat!

- 1 ½ cups pecans
- 12 Medjool dates, pitted, halved
- ¼ tsp salt
- 1 tsp vanilla extract
- ½ cup dark chocolate chips, melted for coating
- sprinkles, optional

In a food processor, pulse the first four ingredients until crumbly and then turn the machine on until it all comes together in a big clump. Roll in balls and place on a cookie sheet. Set in the freezer while you are melting the dipping chocolate. Using a double boiler (a large glass bowl on top of a small pot of simmering water), add the chocolate chips to the bowl until melted, stirring frequently. Once melted, drop one ball at a time using a fork to gently turn to coat and lift out. If you want to use the sprinkles, sprinkle them over the ball when it comes out of the chocolate. Place back on a cookie sheet to place in the freezer or refrigerator until hardened. Store in the refrigerator or freezer.

Makes about 20 cookie dough balls.

Peanut Butter Bites

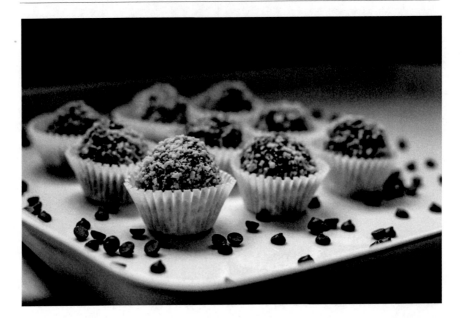

My sons love these even with the dates left out, but you may need to work your way up to that if you are used to the sweetness of candy bars.

Coating:

- ½ cup salted peanuts
- ¼ cup unsweetened shredded coconut.

Filling:

- 1 cup salted peanuts
- ¾ cup dark chocolate chips
- 15 Medjool dates, pitted, halved (optional)
- 1 tsp pure vanilla extract
- 2 T almond butter

Make the coating first by processing the peanuts and shredded coconut until crumbly. Set aside in a bowl. For the filling, process the peanuts and chocolate chips together until a fine crumble; add the dates until mixed in; add the remaining ingredients and keep the machine running until the mixture starts to stick to itself. Roll into balls and then roll into the coating.

Refrigerate until ready to eat. Makes about 15 balls.

Chocolate Almond Bites

When you are craving something sweet, this should do the trick.

- 6 Medjool dates, pitted, halved
- ¾ cup unsweetened shredded coconut flakes
- ¼ cup dark chocolate chips
- 2 T slivered almonds

Process all ingredients together until batter is sticky enough to roll into balls.

Makes about 12 balls.

Pumpkin Pie

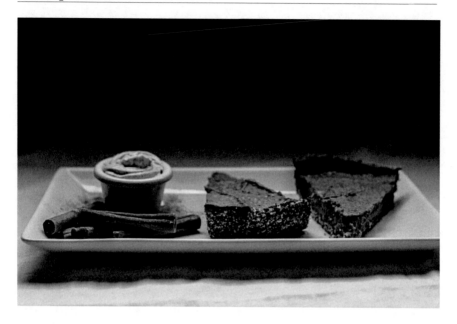

Some say this is better than the real deal. Vanilla bean cream recipe to follow. Find the canned coconut cream at Trader Joe's, various markets, and amazon.com. You could use full fat, canned, coconut milk for this recipe if you can't find the cream.

Crust:

- 1 cup rolled oats
- 3 Medjool dates, pitted, halved
- ½ cup walnuts or pecans
- 1 T water
- Melted coconut oil for greasing pie pan

Preheat oven to 350°F. Lightly grease a 9-inch pie dish with melted coconut oil (dip a napkin in the oil and smear around pan). Process the oats into a flour; add the dates and process until mixed in well. Next, add the nuts and keep the machine running until you notice the oils in the nuts moistening the mixture. Then, add the water. Continue to mix together using the processor. The dough should stick together when pinched. If not, process a little longer. Press into pie dish and poke holes using a fork for venting. Bake crust for 10 minutes. Set aside.

Pumpkin Pie Filling:

- 15 Medjool dates, pitted, halved
- ½ tsp salt
- 1 tsp cinnamon
- ½ tsp ground ginger
- ¼ tsp ground cloves
- 2 T ground flax seed
- 1 can pumpkin puree
- 1 can coconut cream

In a food processor, add the dates and the dry ingredients. Pulse together until the dates are broken up, then turn the machine on until pureed. Transfer to a blender and add the pumpkin puree and coconut cream. Pour into the baked pie shell. Take a piece of tin foil large enough to go under the pie dish and come up around the sides to cover the crust to prevent burning.

Bake at 350°F for about an hour. When the pie is done, let cool and keep in the refrigerator. Serves 8.

Vanilla Bean Cream

My new favorite ingredient for baking is ground vanilla (from the whole bean), also known as vanilla powder. The vanilla taste is so much more intense—especially since it doesn't have the added alcohol. You could substitute it with pure vanilla extract, but you won't get the same depth of flavor. You won't be disappointed splurging on the vanilla powder to have on hand, which can be used in recipes as the same measurements as the extract. I was introduced to the ground vanilla by my sister who surprised me with a package in the mail containing this stuff. What a nice gift! This vanilla bean cream can be used alongside my pumpkin pie or sweet potato pie. You can find it on amazon.com.

- 1 can coconut cream, refrigerated, cream top only
- ½ tsp vanilla powder
- Pinch of freshly ground nutmeg
- 1-2 T maple syrup

The coconut cream needs to be cold in order to scoop out all of the cream. If you shake the can and you hear sloshing around then it's not separated yet and needs to be chilled for a couple of hours. There will be a thin liquid on the bottom of the can that is not used for this recipe. In a medium-sized bowl, scoop out the solidified coconut cream, whisk in the vanilla powder, nutmeg and maple syrup. If the mixture is runny, chill in the refrigerator for a couple of hours until it thickens up. Put a dollop of the cream on top of the pie of your choice. Store in the refrigerator.

Sweet Potato Pie

When I was surrounded by a huge dessert table at Thanksgiving sweet potato pie wasn't something that grabbed me amongst all the other overly sweetened stuff. But this one I'll gravitate towards.

Prep ahead:

- Roasted yams, enough for two cups pureed. (depending on the size 2-6)

Crust:

- 2/3 cup rolled oats
- 1/4 cup pecans
- 6 Medjool dates, pitted, halved
- 1 tsp ground flax seed
- 1/4 tsp baking powder
- 1/4 tsp cinnamon
- 1/4 tsp vanilla extract
- 1/4 cup coconut oil, melted

Filling:

- 10 Medjool dates, pitted, halved
- 2 cups roasted yam puree
- 1/2 cup unsweetened almond milk
- 1/2 tsp ground ginger
- 1/2 tsp ground cinnamon
- 1/8 tsp ground nutmeg
- Pinch ground cloves

For the crust, in a food processor, grind the rolled oats and pecans until flour-like; add the dates and pulse until mixture is sandy. Pulse in the flax seed, baking powder, and cinnamon just to combine. While processor is running, add the coconut oil and vanilla until the dough sticks together when pinched. Press dough onto a pie pan. Set aside.

For the filling, process the dates by themselves until broken up (it's okay if they become a big ball). Add in the yam puree and process to combine, then add remaining ingredients. Pour into pie crust. Keep in the refrigerator. The pie may look like it is not sliceable, but it is. Top with a dollop of vanilla bean cream before serving a slice.

Serves 8.

Fudge Frosting

This is so delicious eaten straight up, or spread on the Flourless Chocolate Brownies (recipe to follow).

- 10 Medjool dates, pitted, halved
- ½ can lite coconut milk
- 1 T coconut oil
- 1 T pure maple syrup
- 1 tsp vanilla extract
- ½ tsp instant coffee
- ¼ cup cocoa powder
- ¼ cup dark chocolate chips

Put the first four ingredients into a sauce pan, and bring to a simmer for about 6 minutes. Remove from the heat, and add the remaining ingredients. Transfer to the food processor and cover the machine with a towel to avoid scalding splashes, or covering your counter in a new shade of brown. Or, let cool on the stove, then transfer. Pulse until smooth. Spread over cooled Flourless Chocolate Brownies, or put in bowl and eat by the spoonful.

Makes about 1 ½ cups.

Flourless Chocolate Brownies

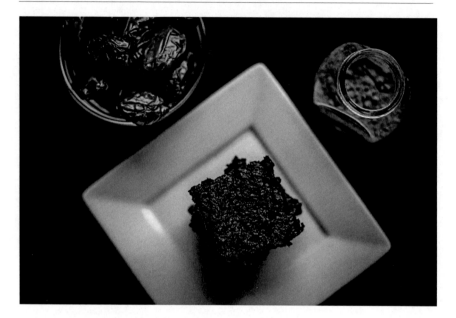

This recipe will win over any health food skeptic.

- 20 Medjool dates, pitted , halved
- 1/2 cup cocoa powder
- 1 cup almond meal
- 1 tsp baking powder
- 1 tsp baking soda
- 1 T ground flax seed
- 1 cup hot water
- 1 tsp vanilla extract
- 1/4 cup coconut oil, melted, plus additional for greasing the pan
- 1/2 cup dark chocolate chips, optional

In a food processor, add the dates with the cocoa powder until chopped up pretty fine; add the almond meal to combine. Pulse in the baking powder, baking soda, and flax seed; carefully pulse in the hot water with the vanilla. Then, add the coconut oil and pulse to mix in. Pour in the chocolate chips; pulse a few times to combine. Pour the batter into a greased 8-in square pan (grease by dipping a napkin in melted coconut oil and smear around pan).

Bake at 350°F for about 35 minutes. Serves 9.

Brown Rice Pudding

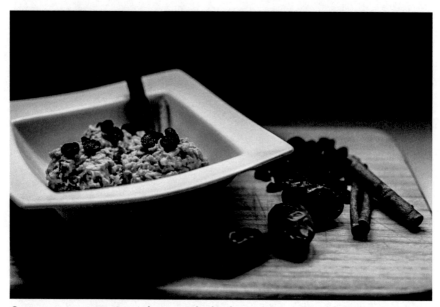

Coconut cream is richer and thicker than most full fat coconut milk and works much better in this recipe. I buy the canned coconut cream at Trader Joe's or you can find on amazon.com.

- 1 cup coconut cream, divided
- 12 Medjool dates, pitted, halved
- 1 tsp vanilla extract
- 2 cups unsweetened almond milk
- 1 tsp cinnamon
- 3 cups cooked, short grain brown rice
- 1/2 cup raisins, optional

In a food processor, pulse ½ of the coconut cream with the dates and vanilla until smooth. Transfer to a bowl; add the remaining coconut cream and almond milk with the cinnamon. Whisk together to combine; add the rice and raisins. Refrigerate until ready to eat. Serves about 6.

Chocolate Ice Cream

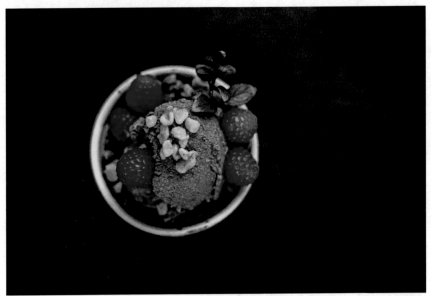

This ice cream rivals the vegan brands sold in the markets only this one does not have sugar. Try it topped with walnuts and raspberries.

- 1 cup cocoa powder
- 23 Medjool dates, pitted, halved
- 1 can coconut cream or can of full fat coconut milk
- 1 ½ cans light coconut milk
- 1 T pure vanilla extract

In a food processor, pulse dates and cocoa powder half at a time to avoid your kitchen being dusted with cocoa powder; pulse until a fine crumble. Transfer to a blender to mix in the remaining ingredients. Next, follow the manufacturer's instructions on your ice cream maker.

Makes about 3 pints.

Peanut Butter Ice Cream

Please don't judge me if you overhear my son say he ate ice cream for breakfast. It is healthier than the majority of cereals out there.

- 1 cup and 2 T natural peanut butter
- 20 Medjool dates, pitted, halved
- 1 can light coconut milk, divided
- 1 can coconut cream or can of full fat coconut milk
- 1 ½ tsp vanilla

In a food processor, add the dates with half of the can of light coconut milk. Transfer to a blender and add the remaining ingredients. Next, follow the manufacturer's instructions on your ice cream maker.

Makes about 3 pints.

Frozen Grasshopper Pie

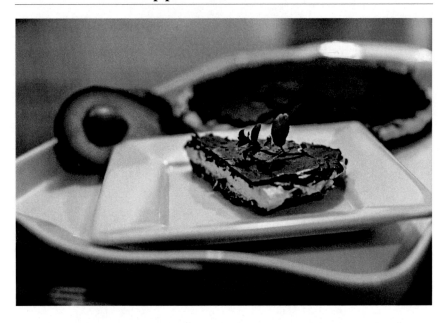

Mmm… chocolate and mint. Maple syrup is the star of this pie. The topping recipe is from a vegan blogger at mydarlingvegan.com. I've also used this topping to dip frozen banana slices in and refroze!

Crust:

- 1 cup slivered almonds
- ¼ cup cocoa powder
- 2 T maple syrup
- 1 tsp peppermint extract

In a food processor, pulse the almonds and cocoa powder together. Add the liquids. Press into the bottom of a spring form pan (or regular pie dish if you don't have a spring form pan). Set aside.

Filling:

- 1 can coconut cream
- 1 avocado, mashed
- 1 tsp vanilla
- 1 tsp mint
- ½ cup maple syrup

Pour all of the ingredients into a blender (a food processor can't handle all of the liquid). When blended, pour over crust and freeze for about two hours.

Topping:

- 1/3 cup coconut oil, melted
- 1 tsp pure vanilla extract
- ¼ cup pure maple syrup
- ¼ cup cocoa powder

Whisk topping ingredients together in a bowl until combined and evenly pour over the top of the frozen grasshopper pie. This will harden immediately on contact. Return to the freezer if you are not eating soon. If this pie is frozen solid allow for about 30 minutes of thaw time at room temperature before serving. Keep in the freezer.

Serves 8.

Extra Dark Fudge Popsicles

If you don't have an ice cream maker, then popsicles are the next best thing. This recipe is good for using up any leftover coconut cream.

- 11 Medjool dates, pitted, halved
- 1/4 cup cocoa powder
- 1/2 tsp pure vanilla extract
- 1 cup unsweetened almond milk
- 1/3 cup can of coconut cream or full fat coconut milk

Place dates, cocoa powder, and vanilla into the bowl of the food processor. Process the dates until broken up. Add the almond milk and coconut cream. For this recipe, it's okay if some of the thinner liquid from the can of coconut milk is mixed in (other recipes require the cream top only formed from the can being chilled). Process until smooth. Pour into four popsicle molds; freeze. To unmold the popsicles, run warm water over the molds to loosen.

Makes 4.

Virgin Margarita Pops

Refreshing! This is not a recipe for true vegans since it contains honey. Make the Extra Dark Fudge Popsicles next to use up the leftover coconut cream.

- zest of two limes
- 1 cup lime juice (about 6 large limes)
- 1 cup coconut cream from a can, shaken.
- 1/2 cup honey

Whisk all together in a bowl until the honey is incorporated. Pour into popsicle molds; freeze. To unmold the popsicles, run warm water over the molds to loosen.

Makes 4-5.

References

Ansel, K. (2015 May/June). Don't have a cow. *Eating Well,* 23.

Estabrook, B. (2015, July/August). Good seed, bad seed. *Eating Well,* 78-86.

Fife, B. (2004). *The coconut oil miracle.* New York: Avery.

Food and Drug Administration. 2003. *Guidance for industry: Trans fatty acids in nutrition labeling, nutrient content claims, health claims; small entity compliance guide.* Retrieved June 23, 2015, from https://www.fda.gov/food/guidanceregulatio n/guidancedocumentsregulatoryinformation/ucm053479.ht m.

Harper, B. (2014). *Skinny meals.* New York: Ballantine Books.

Lanzisera, F. (2015, Jan/Feb). Food sensitivities and weight gain. *Simply Gluten Free,* 32.

mydarlingvegan.com. (2013, Jan 13). *Raw chocolate hazelnut cheesecake.* Retrieved from: http://mydarlingvegan.com/ 2013/01/raw-chocolate-hazelnut-cheesecake/

Petersen, V. (2015, Jan/Feb). Gluten and dairy: The undeniable connection. *Simply Gluten Free,* 45.

Quillin, P. (2005). *Beating cancer with nutrition* (4th ed.). Nutrition Times Press: Carlsbad.

thediva-dish.com. (2012, April 2). *Sugar free chocolate chip bean cookies and homemade date puree.* Retrieved from: http://thediva-dish.com/desserts/sugar-free-chocolate-chip-bean-cookies-and-homemade-date-puree/

Warner, M. (2013). *Pandora's lunchbox.* New York: Scribner

Made in the USA
San Bernardino, CA
19 March 2016